Dr. John Sarno's Top 10 Healing Discoveries

Steve Ozanich

Foreword by
Andrea Leonard-Segal, MD

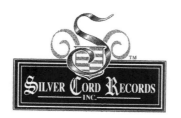

SILVER CORD RECORDS
INC.

Disclaimer:

This book contains medical and psychological information relating to health care. It is not intended to be a supplement for medical or psychological treatment or evaluation. It is strongly recommended that you seek professional advice regarding your health before attempting to incorporate into your life any advice enclosed. Therefore, both the publisher and the author should not be held responsible for any medical outcomes that may result from utilizing the methods contained or suggested in this book. Exhaustive efforts have been made to secure the accuracy of the information contained within this book—as of first publication.

ISBN: 978-0-9965866-1-0

First Edition

Designed by Steve Ozanich

Cover layout and design: Taylor Krzeszowski

Publisher: Silver Cord Records, Inc.

PO Box 8513
Warren, OH 44484

SteveOzanich.com

Printed on acid-free paper

For Doctor Sarno

You changed the world...
but the world doesn't know it yet.

Contents

Foreword

Dr. Sarno's work on mindbody healing, while a Professor of Rehabilitation Medicine at New York University Medical Center, changed countless lives for the better with lasting effects. He was a brilliant, observant, and caring physician who was courageous enough to see chronic pain in a completely new way and to change the way it was diagnosed and treated. Over the past 50 years, he has helped at minimum tens of thousands of people to heal, thousands who were lucky enough to see him as patients in his office, and vast, incalculable numbers of patients who benefitted from reading one of his four books on the diagnosis and treatment of chronic pain that are published worldwide in multiple languages. Even though Dr. Sarno has now retired from his medical practice, he continues to regularly receive correspondence from new patients who have recently read one of his books on the condition that he calls the Tension Myoneural Syndrome (TMS) and have felt compelled to express their endless gratitude to him for bringing them back to health.

I am a physician, board certified in internal medicine and rheumatology, in practice at the George Washington University Center for Integrative Medicine and on the clinical faculty at the George Washington University School of Medicine and Health Sciences. It was my honor to have collaborated with Dr. Sarno professionally for more than 25 years. I was thrilled when Columbia University Medical Center asked me to make a presentation honoring Dr. Sarno's work at a conference on psychosomatic medicine that was held in January of 2016. This public recognition of the major impact that Dr. Sarno's work has made on health care is long overdue.

Dr. Sarno was my wisest and best mentor and is a dear friend. In my own medical practice, I have treated patients from all over the world and all over the United States, who have traveled far distances to find a cure for their pain. Before I understood Dr. Sarno's work and how to diagnose and treat patients with TMS, I was making the "usual" diagnoses that physicians make and prescribing the "standard care" treatments to help patients with chronic musculoskeletal pain syndromes like common back and neck pain, fibromyalgia, rotator cuff syndrome, carpal tunnel syndrome, etc. These "standard care" treatments (e.g., some pain medications, back surgery, physical therapy) were not well validated by well-conducted clinical trials in the medical literature. Despite this, they were, and still are, widely recommended by many well-intended physicians and other healthcare professionals who are, unfortunately, not able to understand or are not interested in the impact of the mind on the well-being of the body. Once I understood the underlying psychological etiology of these conditions and started making the TMS diagnosis and using a psychological approach to treatment, my ability to help my patients soared.

Any patient who is not feeling well should see a physician to be sure that there is nothing serious causing the problem. Once serious conditions, such as cancer, infection, or fracture are ruled out, it is important to consider whether psychological factors could be responsible for the physical symptoms.

Steve Ozanich, a former back pain patient who suffered for years while receiving the "usual diagnoses and treatments," ultimately healed because of Dr. Sarno's discoveries. In this book, he has succinctly captured many of the principles that Dr. Sarno taught to patients. This is a small book with a big message.

Andrea Leonard-Segal, MD, FACR
January 21, 2016

Introduction

When I was first introduced to Dr. John Sarno's work in the mid-1990s, I rejected it forthwith. Like the majority of those who cannot come to accept it, I didn't understand it, and hadn't grown tired enough of my suffering to listen. Now, two decades later I teach the work to others.

Daily, I educate suffering individuals on exactly what the good doctor's oeuvre is about. I have been witness to those aspects of his work that have been the most helpful in healing; those ideas that have risen to the forefront in their impact on public awareness, and therefore healing.

In this book, I have ordered those concepts into a list of insights that I have observed make the most powerful impact. Even though it is impossible to assign numerical values to psychological concepts, this "top 10" catalogue of breakthrough discoveries is changing lives every day. The purpose of the list itself is to pull together a very complex body of work into an easily readable and understandable form. Within greater understanding comes healing.

The core of Dr. Sarno's original body of work has been distorted, spun, and diluted in many cleverly marketable ways by those who don't clearly understand it, who do not make appropriate attribution, and who are seeking to profit materially from Dr. Sarno's work. The spin, which masquerades as "newest" insights and revelations on the work are not new at all and, in fact, have tended to focus on the physical arena once again. This is a terrible shame because Dr. Sarno's discoveries into mindbody medicine are unparalleled as was his ability to successfully diagnose and treat his patients. Nonetheless, his work remains at the cutting edge of understanding and will be for some time.

Here is the heart of what the good doctor revealed to the world.

Dr. John Sarno's Top 10 Observations

 If they can't see it under a microscope, (to them) it doesn't exist.

John Sarno, MD, ABC 20/20, "Dr. Sarno's Cure"

In my mind's eye, I can still see pages of *Healing Back Pain* flying from their cover, as I threw the book against the fireplace above me—paper scattering to the floor where I was lying, in severe pain. I had a pretty good arm back then. I was also more foolish in those days. I had rejected what could have saved me from great agony, choosing the hard road over truth. However, the best thing I ever did for myself was to piece that book back together, and begin to read again with an open mind.

I had the same initial reaction to Dr. Sarno's work that many sufferers do. I felt that it didn't apply to me—that it was nonsense! I had to get much worse before I would finally listen, and then heal. It wasn't so much about putting his book back together, as it was about putting my life back together.

I needlessly suffered through pain for 30 years. When it finally became unbearable, I was forced into seeing deeper. Today I'm free. If I hadn't gotten dramatically worse I would never have healed. As with many former sufferers, I chose to stay in pain until I couldn't tolerate it any more. People will limp around, bend gingerly, move differently, limit themselves in activity, and repeatedly visit doctors, rather than to accept healing. Thanks to Dr. John Sarno, we now know why.

The wisdom of Dr. Sarno's work on mindbody healing, and his courage, changed my life forever. I'm forever thankful to him for standing up for truth in the face of cynical criticism, bursts of outrage, and hatred. He was a medical pioneer in mindbody healing, paving a new trail for others to follow. But I'm not alone in my admiration. As a physician, he improved the lives of people from every walk of life. He was also a doctor's doctor, literally. Doctors went to see him for help with their pain, and he didn't disappoint.

I believe it's conservatively safe to say that he helped millions of people to heal if you consider the millions of copies of his books that have sold, in 16 different languages. Plus, as anyone knows, once the book is purchased, and the person heals, the book get passed around to several more people because many people won't spend $12 for something that will end their suffering. I loaned out my copies of his books to dozens of people who benefited greatly from them. So, the "number of healed" can never be known; but the impact is clear. He changed the world, but the world doesn't know it yet.

Sadly—as with any new revelation—his message came with a cost. The cost was resistance, ridicule, and inexplicable controversy. But his personal rewards far outweighed the professional cost. His reward was seeing people heal, virtually every single time. Sufferers came from everywhere, after trying everything, with no hope, and they healed. German philosopher Arthur Schopenhauer reportedly said, "All truth passes through three stages. First, it is ridiculed, second it is violently opposed, and third, it is accepted as self-evident." The future of Dr. Sarno's work is bright—beyond the resistance.

At the beginning of 2016, his work is beginning to move from the ridicule stage, toward stronger opposition. But without doubt, what he has brought to the public eye will someday be accepted as self-evident. All that's needed is for ignorance to run its course, and to yield to what already is. However, between now and acceptance is lengthy debating yet to be fully engaged.

The resistance to his message is scattered in illogic; much of its impetus drawn from "science blindness." Many people only believe what numbers tell them. To them, nothing can ever be true unless science says it is. But clinical trials can only measure cause and effect. They can't measure reasons, beliefs, motivations, or hope. Too many sufferers hold tight to their personal agony by hiding behind **science as a psychological defense mechanism**. They often do this by coming up with resistance statements to Dr. Sarno's work using a "lack of science" as a shield to avoid healing.

Common defense mechanisms include:

- Where are the numbers?
- Science doesn't support it!
- Everyone is different; what works for one person may not work for another.
- Dr. Sarno's work is okay, but it didn't work for me.
- Did anger make my back disc herniate?
- That's stupid, my body makes noises!
- My pain is real…!!!
- I was in an accident; no one is going to tell me my pain is all in my head!!
- Dr. Sarno doesn't know what pain is or he would never say such things!

Such statements defend suffering. Even worse—none of them is true, for different and varying reasons. The primary reason that these statements are false, itself explains why they're all false—and that reason is that these people don't know what they're talking about. But I can understand their resistance because I initially reacted the same way.

 People are doing the best that they can from their own level of consciousness.

Deepak Chopra, MD

Dr. Sarno never said the pain wasn't real. In fact, he said it was the most painful thing he had ever seen in clinical medicine. His work has nothing to do with injuries, so why would anyone bring up accidents as a resistance statement? Back pain doesn't come from herniated discs so the anger/herniation straw man can't stand up on its own. And body noises don't cause pain. The above statements are all false, which is why these people don't understand TMS, and are still in pain.

Statements such as, "I tried Dr. Sarno's quackery but it didn't work!!" is a gross misunderstanding of his work, and the process. It simply doesn't happen that way. You have to fully accept the truth, invest in it 100%, and then get down and begin the life-transforming work. **You have to want to heal**. Healing has nothing to do with getting rid of pain. Healing is about taking away the **need** for the pain—its cause. By removing the cause, you remove the effect, which is the pain itself.

Perhaps the worst resistance statement comes from suggesting that Dr. Sarno doesn't know what pain is. He, too, suffered from many types of pain, and overcame them. He understands.

The naysayers hear part of the message, and draw an entire universe of wrong conclusions, as they fight to hold onto their symptoms—much like a fool throwing a book at a fireplace. Poor understanding, fueled by ulterior motives, leads to erroneous conclusions drawn from false assumptions. Another culprit is the wild-west Internet where anyone can say anything, about anybody—true or untrue.

Healing requires that truth itself be desired, rigorously sought—and eventually accepted. Anyone who wants to heal will look closely at Dr. Sarno's work. It is effective—virtually every single time. The demand for more proof, and more science, and more numbers is a shield against the unwanted. Resistance allows those who are suffering to blame something else beyond their control—to escape the true cause of their suffering. Incredulously, if shown a study to support Dr. Sarno's findings, they will often state, "But was it a double blind trial?" Then—if shown a double blind, they will often respond with things like, "Oh yeah? But what about this and what about that?" No amount of evidence will ever be enough for someone who needs to protect their pain. The **reason this controversy is significant** is that the reason they reject the cure ... is the very reason they have their pain.

This was a landmark discovery of Dr. Sarno. Very few are aware enough to see it, and fewer are brave enough to admit it. But for those who are ready to end their suffering, his work is heaven-sent. As the aphorism states, "Pain is inevitable, suffering is a choice." It's not about whether the processes Dr. Sarno described work or not, because they do; it's a matter of understanding, and acceptance.

> There is lots of research [on mindbody healing]. It's published in bona-fide and major medical journals, but it disappears without trace. It's like it has no impact on practice. It's DESPITE the evidence, not for the lack of it, that we practice the way we do.
>
> Gabor Mate, MD, author of *When the Body Says No*

Why would anyone reject something that could take away pain? **The pain exists to protect them from deeper aspects of themselves—to bury the truth.** So, rejection makes perfect sense! Why would anyone want to take away something that's protecting them? When shown information that can take suffering away, why is the first reaction, "That's stupid!" Why isn't the first reaction, "Show me how!" This controversy is at the heart of the story of pain.

> I believe that all medical studies are flawed if they do not consider the emotional factor.
>
>   John Sarno, MD, *Healing Back Pain*, p. 147

We can't measure love, despair, laughter, sadness, or hope. But we know they exist. We also know that healing happens outside the measurable realm, where the real person lives—within the unconscious. Science doesn't reveal Truth; it often distorts it. People are emotional beings, and the impact of emotions on health can't be measured. Dr. Sarno found the magic bullet in healing—**belief**. People who believe their body is broken remain in pain. Those who believe their body is okay, tend to heal. The only thing that matters is results, and Dr. Sarno certainly achieved them.

John E. Sarno, MD, is the greatest pain doctor who has ever lived, a pioneering pain physician. But his work goes well beyond understanding pain. It unveiled the intricacies that define the many causes that give rise to epidemics of suffering. He not only identified and verbalized the many elements and contributing factors that cause pain—but also, the causes and effects adding to overall health problems.

His 50-year career as a physician was defined by his discovery of **TMS**. It was the centerpiece of his life. In the early years, the acronym, TMS, came from the phrase, **Tension Myositis Syndrome**, and evolved to the term **Tension Myoneural Syndrome**, and finally to **The Mindbody Syndrome**. As he learned more, the term morphed to define the discoveries better.

Truth isn't expanding; our awareness of it is.

Within his discovery of TMS, he observed many other phenomena that contributed to his becoming an historic healer. He accomplished this through **observation**. He learned how to help people heal themselves, by listening to them.

In today's world of health and healing, much has gone wrong, and more is misunderstood. She is more than her pain. He is more than his physical body. Each sufferer comes into the doctor's office with a life of emotions, and relationships—with a past. Every individual's body reacts strongly to fear, anger, resentment, sadness, anxiety, guilt, and shame that are created by conflicted thoughts. Dr. Sarno put the patient back into the healing equation, driven by the thirst for truth, light. Pioneers don't follow, they lead—supported by few. There were no Forewords in Dr. Sarno's books.

I spent 10 years researching and writing *The Great Pain Deception*. I've also been consulting, talking to, and helping people with TMS for over 16 years. I've witnessed people healing from many types of health problems, in many countries, using Dr. Sarno's work. It's been highly rewarding to be part of such a great movement, and to help people through education. I've noted along the way just how many great observations Dr. Sarno actually had, and how those observations are now healing people, every day, in dramatic ways.

He's become known by those who have healed as the **good doctor**. However, his insights were so profound that it doesn't seem right to call him a good doctor, but rather he is a **great doctor**. The following are what I believe to be his top 10 discoveries of observation.

#10

Many Surgeries for Pain Are Placebos

Placebos take many forms: surgery, a variety of other physical treatments, and pharmaceuticals. If the celestial architect were to suddenly abolish the placebo effect in humans, there would be economic chaos, particularly in the United States for much medical treatment today owes its success … to the placebo phenomenon.

John Sarno, MD, *The Divided Mind,* p. 31

We can easily look at the great doctor's successful body of work, along with the newer placebo trials, and see that most of the back surgeries, knee, hand, foot, neck, and shoulder surgeries have done little or nothing, over the past 100 years. With great hindsight, prompted by great insight—we can now see how the sufferers' beliefs had healed them, rarely the surgery itself. This holds true for most therapeutic modalities like chiropractic, acupuncture, joint renewal products, core alignment, and core strengthening, etc. … the truth is being slowly exposed by the many placebo trials that, unfortunately, are for the most part disregarded by both the medical industry and the general population.[1]

Proof of Nothing

In the 1950s, researchers wondered if the technique of tying off damaged arteries (internal mammary ligation) was any better than doing nothing at-all for heart patients. So the curious scientists prepared two independent studies in two US cities to try to understand what was really happening. They had been having great

---

[1] I realize the hypocrisy in using science to show how science isn't telling the whole truth. But, when you're trying to explain something to someone, it's best to use the language that the person speaks.

success with the ligation surgeries in heart patients, but they wanted to know if what they were doing was actually doing anything. To test the success, they created two groups. One group got the real ligation surgery and the other got a sham surgery where the participants had an incision in their chest but were sewn up with no ligation. The end results were that the group that had nothing done to them had greater improvement (83%) compared to the group that had the actual surgery (67%).[2] The "successful" ligation surgeries had been doing nothing all along. The patients' belief that it was working made it work.

Other studies continuously prove this same concept. Parkinson's patients who thought they had received embryonic stem cells began feeling better, but they had received fake surgery. One woman, who was inactive due to her Parkinson's symptoms, began ice skating and hiking after she received sham surgery.[3]

Placebo researcher, Ted Kaptchuk, OMD, reported that during his placebo trials, people given fake acupuncture developed raised red bumps where the acupuncture needles were inserted, but no needles ever penetrated the skin. Other participants involved in placebo pain pill trials, who hoped to reduce arm pain, carpal tunnel, elbow pain, shoulder, tendinitis, and wrist pain through use of the pills, reported feeling poorly, and sluggish—even having trouble getting out of bed. However, no pain pills were ever given; they received only cornstarch.[4]

---

[2] EG Diamond, CF Kittle, JE Crockett, "Comparison of Internal Mammary Artery Ligation and Sham Operation for Angina Pectoris," American Journal of Cardiology, vol. 5, no. 4, pp. 483-486 (1960).
LA Cobb, GI Thomas, DH Dillard, et al, An Evaluation of Internal Mammary Artery Ligation by a Double Blind Technic," NEJM, vol.260 no. 22, pp. 1115-1118 (1959).
[3] http://www.medicalnewstoday.com/releases/7100.php
[4] Psychology of Pain, Gary B. Rollman, Emeritus Professor of Psychology, University of Western Ontario, 12/24/12.

A March 2015 study, published in The Clinical Journal of Pain[5] on the effects of acupuncture, concluded that the success of acupuncture depended on the sufferer's expectations of it. If the sufferer believed it would work, it had better results. Those who didn't have much belief had little improvement. The same is true for surgery and most other medical procedures. The only benefits come from the patient's attitude and expectations. Lead author on the 2015 study, Felicity Bishop, PhD, stated, "People who started out with very low expectations of acupuncture–who thought it probably would not help them–were more likely to report less benefit as treatment went on."

> This study emphasizes the influence of the placebo effect on pain.
>
> Stephen Simpson, PhD, Director of Research
> at Arthritis Research UK

In 2002, the Baylor College of Medicine conducted a knee surgery trial on diseased knees using arthroscopy, and discovered that osteoarthritis (the most common type of degenerative joint disease) of the knee heals just as well if fake surgery is performed.[6] Nelda Wray, MD, lead investigator of this study stated, "The fact that the effectiveness of arthroscopic lavage or debridement in patients with osteoarthritis of the knee is no greater than that of placebo surgery makes us question whether the dollars spent on these procedures might not be put to better use."

---

[5] "Psychological Covariates of Longitudinal Changes in Back-related Disability in Patients Undergoing Acupuncture," Bishop, Felicity L. PhD; Yardley, Lucy PhD,; Prescott, Philip PhD; Cooper, Cyrus MA, DM, FRCP, FMedSci; Little, Paul MD, PhD, FRCGP; Lewith, George T. MA, MD, FRCP, MRCGP, The Clinical Journal of Pain, March 2015 - Volume 31 - Issue 3 - p 254–264.

[6] B. Moseley et al. "A Controlled Trial of Arthroscopic Surgery for Osteoarthritis of the Knee," New England Journal of Medicine 2002; 347: 81-8.

> I hate to tell you this, but surgery may have the biggest placebo effect of all.
>
> Nelda Wray, MD, MPH, Professor of Medicine, Division of Preventive Medicine, University of Alabama School of Medicine

Bruno Klopfer, PhD, reported on a patient with lymph node cancer who had been treated with an experimental drug called Krebiozen. The man recovered from many of his many large tumors, and was doing well until he heard that Krebiozen wasn't any good. From that point he got worse, and returned to the state he was in prior to the administration of the drug. Klopfer then told the patient that he would give him a stronger form of Krebiozen, but he gave the man sterile water instead. The man's tumors once again disappeared, because he had a deep belief that he was being given a stronger drug. However, once the AMA officially announced its decision that Krebiozen "was of no value," his tumors returned and the man died soon after.

Vertebroplasty is a type of cement injected into discs to heal cracked vertebrae in the spine. It had been performed "successfully" in more than a million people. However, the technique's creators had noted that there were times that the cement was injected into the wrong disc, and yet the sufferers healed anyway. So they set up a trial to examine the phenomenon and discovered that the people healed the same whether they got the cement, or received nothing at all.

> ... there was no statistically significant difference in improvement in function between the patients who underwent vertebroplasty and placebo.
>
> David Kallmes, MD, Mayo Clinic, study designer

Time and time again—through increased awareness and closer observation—it becomes more obvious that commonly accepted medical techniques have been doing little to nothing. In many cases, the relief begins before the treatments are even administered. The power of belief is immeasurable—and currently, people believe in drugs and surgery. Dr. Gabor Mate is right: there's plenty of evidence to show that these treatments aren't doing anything, but the evidence gets lost without a trace, and has no impact on medical practice. People prefer to get medicalized.

Placebo studies have been around for a long time, but it was Dr. Sarno who once again opened the public eye. He rekindled the fires by shedding new light on the topic of placebo and surgery in his books, *Healing Back Pain*, *The Mindbody Prescription*, and *The Divided Mind*.

Spinal disc surgery is not a panacea for back pain, but the procedure continues every day because surgeons keep doing it, and sufferers keep accepting it.[7] Discectomies are not needed in almost all cases, and often a positive outcome can be the result of the awesome power of **satisfied belief**, through the placebo/healing phenomenon. Dr. Sarno proved it with the tens of thousands of people he helped to heal without surgery, after they had been told they needed discectomies to heal.

The Latin word placebo means, "I shall please." The *surgery pleases the sufferer*, who deeply believes that the surgery and surgeon will help—and so they do. Many people feel post-surgical relief because they are removed from their tension-infested environment, and then have time to recover—which they would have done anyway, without surgery. This applies to almost all pain, from head to toe.

---

[7] Of course there can be extremely rare cases where surgery is needed. Anything is possible. But generally speaking, herniated discs do not cause back pain. Those who feel their spine is the exception are almost always utilizing a defense mechanism, and any positive outcome from surgery, fusion, or therapy results only from deep belief.

And now—with Dr. Sarno's astronomical successes—Pandora's Box has been thrown wide open, placing into question the true outcomes of many types of surgeries, and numerous other therapeutic procedures. People are fooled into thinking a procedure has worked because of their own **belief**; mingled with the complex interactions of *ego, placebo*, and *symptom equivalency shifting*.

The closer we look, the more steadily the picture comes into focus. But you can't focus anything unless you can see that it's out of focus. Dr. Sarno refocused the picture: most surgeries and medical procedures are placebos. But the concept isn't new. Brilliant people have observed the phenomenon for centuries.

> One of the most successful physicians I have ever known, has assured me, that he used more bread pills, drops of colored water, and powders of hickory ashes, than of all other medicines put together. It was certainly a pious fraud. But the adventurous physician goes on, and substitutes presumption for knowledge ... the patient, treated on the fashionable theory, sometimes gets well in spite of the medicine.
>
> Thomas Jefferson, letter to Dr. Caspar Wistar,
> June 21, 1807

#9

Physicophobia

One must confront TMS, fight it, or the symptoms will continue.

John Sarno, MD, *Healing Back Pain*, p. 81

Physicophobia is Dr. Sarno's "fear of physical activity," as a more effective distractor than the pain itself. The fear of movement shields the pain by protecting it, preventing healing. If you are afraid to pick up your child, or to sit in a chair, or to exercise, then that fear itself does a better job in helping you avoid the emotions behind your pain than does the experience (sensation) of pain itself.

Most pain practitioners tell sufferers to "be careful," and "take it easy," because they feel the sufferer's body needs to be babied to prevent further damage. Regarding The Mindbody Syndrome, that advice is making people worse. The great doctor wrote, "The various health disciplines interested in the back have succeeded in creating an army of the partially disabled in this country with their medieval concepts of structural damage and injury as the basis of back pain." He reversed the old paradigm by telling people to become much more aggressive in physical movement because there's nothing wrong with the spine. There's nothing to heal. If the spinal structure is the problem in back pain, then why does the rate of back pain drop off after the age of 50? The problems should worsen with aging, but they don't ... because the structure of the body is not the cause of most pain.

We are far, far, far stronger than we think we are. Our bodies can take much. Unfortunately, the pain industry has brainwashed people into believing they are frail, broken, and in the need of constant repair. Most sufferers believe that to heal they need to protect their body. But the sufferer needs to push his body in order to heal, and to become aware of what's going on psychologically.

Most individuals in chronic pain are well versed in the common protocols of lying around, supported with pillows, bracing—feet elevated, enveloped in comfort, and barricaded with protection. It all makes sense if the body is damaged. But it's also why there are so many epidemics of pain. It's vital to slowly get rid of the fear of structural damage, and the fear of movement.

Physicophobia plays directly into the brain's strategy of deceit. Rigorous physical movement teaches the brain to react differently to movement. It radically reduces fear once the person realizes that movement won't make him worse. The pain may increase in the short run, but in the long run it won't get worse, it will get better. **Fear of movement keeps the pain reoccurring.** This line of thought is counterintuitive to what most understand, but the majority of sufferers benefited from the great doctor's advice. He taught us to challenge our understanding of pain, and to never let it control us.

> I cannot recall one person who has subsequently said that this advice (to become more physical) caused him or her to have further back trouble.

John Sarno, MD, *Healing Back Pain*, p. 80

This applies to every type of TMS pain, from feet and hands, to shoulders and knees, and head to toe. Healing occurs when you can do anything you want to do with little or no pain ... *and* ... when you no longer fear your pain.

It takes confidence—and fear is a lack of confidence. As long as she fears her pain, she will have reoccurrences. Fear must be overcome, and it begins with challenging the fear of movement. This can be done gradually, or aggressively—after initial healing has occurred, and confidence is raised.

#8

Stop All Forms of Treatment

> Another essential for full recovery is that all forms of physical treatment or therapy **must be abandoned** ... patients are usually shocked when it is suggested that they stop the exercises and stretching they have been taught to do ...

John Sarno, MD, *Healing Back Pain,* p. 81

The belief that the physical body is the cause of the pain keeps the sufferer in pain. Therefore, the use of any type of healing modality mistakenly reinforces a belief in the sufferer's mind that the body is somehow "flawed." The concept in healing is to connect the symptoms to the emotions, and to shift awareness away from the body and back to *feeling, activity,* and *purpose*—in **mindfulness.**

Everything the sufferer is doing "to relieve pain" must stop. This includes acupuncture, chiropractic manipulations, physical therapy, stretching, strengthening, surgery, steroid injections, alignment techniques, ointments, braces, shoe lifts, tapping, touching, and tampering. These things are *nocebos.*

Nocebo is a Latin word meaning, "I will harm." The modalities themselves aren't the problem—the problem is in the faulty diagnoses. Since with TMS, nothing is wrong with the body, any healing techniques utilized are dramatically maintaining awareness on the body, and must be stopped. If these things appear to be helping in any way, it is due to the *placebo.*

All the tips and tricks on how to heal pain are making things worse because of the **nocebo effect**—aided by the **archetypal influence** of the professional, and their ill-fated words of advice.

People make the painful error of believing that everything their doctor tells them is true; but regarding TMS pain, almost nothing the health professional tells them is true.

People sometimes get confused and believe they should stop everything. But the only things that need to be stopped are those things intended to heal the body. Things such as massage are okay. Massage does exactly what it's supposed to do—relax and soothe. So massage can be continued as long as it's understood that it's not being performed for healing, but rather for relaxation and tension reduction only. Also, as David Schechter, MD, has stated, it's okay to get a massage, but it's vital to make sure that it's a "silent massage." Masseuses sometimes get in the ill-advised habit of diagnosing people as having bad rotator cuffs, poor alignment, bulging discs, and worn and torn body parts. This makes the problem worse because it reinforces in the sufferer's mind that something is wrong, when there certainly is not. While getting a massage, it's better to talk about the latest baseball scores or something *really* important, like who's hotter, Ginger or Mary Ann?

The same is true for activities like strengthening, and stretching, and yoga, etc. As long as these things are done for their own sake, and for a feeling of overall wellness, they can be continued. The deeper self knows exactly why an activity is being performed; it can't be fooled. Therefore, stop all body-focused healing modalities, but don't stop living, relaxing, laughing, learning, moving, and freeing yourself from fear.

#7

The Brain Will
"Sometimes Use" the Malformations

Spurious: Latin, adjective, *not true; false.*

Correlation: Latin, noun, *a relationship between things that happen together.*

Spurious Correlation: *A wrong assumption that two things are correlated, when they are not. A spurious correlation is the result of a third factor that is not apparently evident at the time of observation.*

Spurious correlations provide worthless information from studies every day. But people love, and demand, studies—despite a lack of meaningful correlation. Studies are too often the processes of chasing truth and distorting it. They rarely uncover the whole truth, but they can provide valuable information if their goal is to seek *aspects of truth*, and not simply to study for study's sake. The problem is in the difficulty in setting up the study. If a study is set up incorrectly, then you get GIGO—garbage in garbage out.

Dr. Sarno made the insightful and courageous statement that, "The brain will sometimes use the malformations in the body," based on his vast experience. These malformations include such conditions as herniated discs, sites of osteoarthritis, wearing and tearing on knee menisci and rotator cuffs, and the highly questionable "bone on bone" diagnosis (which some doubt even exists). He also made the incisive proclamation, "The idea nerves are being pinched is **fantasy**, and once again much ado about nothing." Sometimes a "spinal abnormality" will be on the right side, but the pain will be on the left side. Sometimes the pain will be at a different level than a herniation—and—sometimes the pain will be **right at the same location as the abnormality.** But it still means nothing because of the spurious correlation. The disc bulging isn't the cause of the back or neck pain. The pain is due to oxygen reduction through the autonomic nervous system (ANS). In any spurious relationship, the two events have no direct connection at all, but are wrongly connected together either by coincidence *or* by a hidden third factor known as a "confounding factor." In the case of TMS and most pain, the third factor, which isn't readily observable at the time of examination, is the powerful emotions that are causing imbalance in the autonomic functions.

There are nearly three dozen studies that have shown that spinal disc herniations are only coincidentally at sites of pain—proving Dr. Sarno correct. But few care to hear such conclusions. The herniations by themselves don't cause back pain, but **the brain will sometimes use** malformations such as arthritis, narrowing (stenosis) and degenerations, when it needs to more firmly convince the sufferer that he has a body problem. This includes numerous malformations in the shoulders, knees, hands, feet, hips, and elsewhere. This is a tremendously insightful observation that is at the foundation for understanding healing.

During times of great tension the old sites of injury, or of significant degenerative changes, will often begin to hurt, making the victim of the ruse think they have somehow re-injured themselves, or that the ole' trick knee is suddenly acting up. But that isn't what's really happening. The observant brain is simply looking for a target—and old injury sites are places where it feels there should be an ongoing problem because *it remembers* the old injury. This is an *awareness of the brain to know* where all the changes are occurring, and have occurred. Once again, the proof that these sites are not the causes of pain is that the people regularly heal even though the sites remain "malformed."

TMS physician Marc Sopher, MD, wrote, "Jack was a former athlete, now in his 40s, with left hip pain. His orthopedist told him that he would benefit from a new hip joint as his x-ray showed 'significant' degenerative changes. After this visit, his left hip pain increased and he mentioned it to me at the time of his annual physical exam. When he told me that his right hip felt fine, I asked him to humor me by having both of his hips x-rayed. On x-ray, both hips had the same 'degenerative' changes, yet his right hip did not hurt! I advised him to put off surgery, resume activity and not pay too much attention to his hips. Following these instructions, his discomfort subsided and he successfully resumed exercise and athletics."

The spurious correlation is a major player in the ongoing pain epidemics around the world. Sufferers who have osteophytes (bone spurs), ankle and hip arthritis, spinal disc herniations, and a myriad of other structural changes are routinely told that these things are causing their pain, but they are not, in almost all cases. These things are "incidental to the pain," meaning, they're just there—the brain uses them to target "when needed."

Dr. Sopher, along with many other medical doctors, has stated that things like infections can also be incidental because the medication often takes away the infection, but the problem remains. So things like tension can cause a sore throat, and when the immunity has been compromised the infection sneaks in behind. The infection then gets blamed for the sore throat—but infection was not the cause in many cases, it was a byproduct.

The most common example of this is the ulcer. Almost everyone on planet Earth has the ulcer bacterium in their stomach, but only those under great stress get the ulcer. The stress compromises immunity, allowing the already present bacteria to run rampant. The bacteria did not cause the ulcer; it was an after-effect. The same is true for the spinal disc herniation. The herniations exist but are not the cause of the pain. The herniations themselves are most likely there "pre-injury;" but there was no reason to do imaging prior to the occurrence of pain. Hence, there was no knowledge that the herniation already existed.

Waleed Brinjikji, MD, along with colleagues, conducted meta-analysis of 33 articles on more than 3,100 people with lumbar disc abnormalities, but who had no pain. The scientists stated that the findings of disc degeneration, disc signal loss, disc height loss, disc protrusion, and facet arthropathy are "part of normal aging and not pathologic processes requiring intervention." They concluded, "These findings suggest that many imaging-based degenerative features may be part of normal aging and unassociated with low back pain, especially when incidentally seen."[8]

This, once again, fits perfectly with Dr. Sarno's clinical observations. Pain will go away without any type of intervention, if the sufferer can accept the notion that the pain is *not coming from the changes in the body*. The brain is only **using the body changes** for its purpose. This is an amazing observation.

---

[8] "Systematic Literature Review of Imaging Features of Spinal Degeneration in Asymptomatic Populations," W. Brinjikji, P.H. Luetmer, B. Comstock, B.W. Bresnahan, L.E. Chen, R.A. Deyo, S. Halabi, J.A. Turner, A.L. Avins, K. James, J.T. Wald, D.F. Kallmes and J.G. Jarvik. American Journal of Neuroradiology, November 27, 2014, doi: 10.3174/ajnr.A4173.

#6

The Rage/Soothe Ratio

 Suppose, however, there is another element in the equation; that it is not simply the quantity of rage that brings on symptoms, but the presence or absence of counterbalancing soothing factors … the occurrence of symptoms reflects too much rage and not enough counteracting soothing elements in one's life.

John Sarno, MD, *The Mindbody Prescription*, p. 29

In his third book, the great doctor writes about a **rage-to-soothe ratio**. The idea is that people will naturally have a certain level of stressors, frustrations, resentment, and disappointments, and therefore anger (rage) in their lives. This results from the type of life they have chosen, how they have adapted to react to that life, and of course from any traumas they have experienced along the way.

However, they also may not be receiving enough pleasure, or soothing, to counterbalance their current level of stress and tension. One reason is that they often don't feel worthy of having fun, or being happy, or even loved. They feel that punishment is their due because they have *extreme guilt*, and feel that pleasure and fun are something they don't deserve to experience. If they try to enjoy a situation, their predisposed guilt prevents them from being mindful of the moment. Unworthiness robs them of pleasure, as they look at their watches, and reflect on all they "should be doing" to be a better person. Perfection and control won't allow for joy because the concept of joy is to be in the present, without constraints and parameters. Joy simply is.

Mindbody disorders are forms of self-punishment against rejected self-images. So naturally, sufferers have lowered self-esteem and don't feel justified in seeking pleasure. They've often been criticized and knocked down, and have experienced what Dr. Sarno labeled "subtle abuses." Many loving parents use "humiliation parenting" to get more out of their children by telling them things like, "Why can't you get all 'A's in school like this person or that person?" Or, "You ought to be ashamed of yourself." These parents don't beat the child, but they verbally push them to be more, and better—*something other than themselves*. And conflict is born.

All of these subtle messages are taken by the child as not being good enough. Many end up being great talents, artists and athletes, super employees: very successful, driven people. They overcome low esteem and inferiorities by succeeding. But there's a price for being motivated by shame, and it's the cost of good health.

There are of course the abused and abandoned children who often harbor considerable rage as adults. Their anger is understandable, but it doesn't mean they have to suffer forever, or that they don't deserve pleasure.

Sufferers aren't necessarily overwhelmed by their stress and anger, but they may not be allowing for anywhere near enough fun. They're more often good people with no emotional balance, giving more of themselves than they can possibly give—giving more than they feel they're getting back. The demands they place on themselves in order to be loved and accepted, and to avoid rejection, create a natural amount of stress, and tension (stension). They then often have trouble enjoying what they've already succeeded in accomplishing.

There is bad stress: **distress**; and there is good stress: **eustress**.

"Eu" comes from "euphoric"—a good and healthy stress that is missing in people with chronic illness and pain. Healthy fun stress releases dopamine and oxytocin that make the individual feel good, forcing an overall sense of well-being. Unfortunately, the driven

individual senses *distress* instead of well-being, through faulty
perception. The way in which a person perceives daily events is an
important factor in how their body will respond. Fun stress can
prolong life, as it increases good health and vitality. Distress causes
rage, and all kinds of health issues. The only difference between the
two is in how life-events are perceived. Of course, tragedy is
rightfully perceived as distressful, but all the little points
throughout the day are open to translation. Most people in chronic
pain perceive daily events as distressful, through a false prism.

Learning how to have fun, allowing for joy, and to be
genuinely happy, eases pain by soothing the fires of rage. But
because of guilt, from the **tyranny of the "should,"** people simply
won't allow for fun to enter awareness.

When sufferers use affirmations in healing they often affirm
things like "I am healing" ... or, "My body is healed." These are
good statements that begin to reverse the false notions of a failed
body. However, many gurus of affirmation are telling people to
affirm things like, "I deserve to be loved ... I forgive easily... I have
value ... I have worth." These affirmations are better in healing
because they go more directly to the heart of the problem, which is
the need for the pain. Many sufferers don't feel deserving of joy, and
so pleasure is avoided and replaced with worry. Negative feelings and
emotions need to be countered to create a well-balanced state. When
a person feels worthy, and loved, they will allow themselves to laugh
and to relax—and the body begins to heal.

The maxim states, "Work hard, play hard." It's extremely
common for people to miss a day off, or have to work through their
time off, and then become sick. The great doctor had yet another
tremendous insight by noting that the *presence of symptoms* could
simply be from the *absence of soothers*.

#5

Emotional Barometer

 (But) … the occurrence of an acute spasm means that there has to be something psychological going on because TMS is an emotional barometer.

John Sarno, MD, *Healing Back Pain*, pg. 84

It's very common to hear people say, "Oh, that's not bothering me, I got over that a long time ago" … or… "My life is going well!" However, they aren't aware that there are emotional processes occurring outside of their awareness, 24/7—and that it's all unconscious—they don't sense any sorrow, fear, anger, or frustration.

"Unconscious" means they don't know it. The only ways in which they become aware that these emotions exist is through the unpleasant symptoms. If the person has TMS, or chronic symptoms, they never did "get over it a long time ago," and they don't truly perceive their life as going well, deep within themselves. "It" is still bothering them outside of their **conscious awareness.** They say they aren't bothered, and that they've gotten over everything. But they haven't; it's a **reaction-formation.**

Reaction-formation is a psychological defense mechanism used to protect ego and to reduce anxiety. Ego attempts to avoid shame by pretending to adhere to the opposite impulse by distorting the unwanted unconscious impulses into a socially acceptable form. In other words, people sometimes behave in an opposite manner to hide their true feelings. E.g., if someone hates someone, and may want to kill them, they may become overly nice to that person to hide the objectionable impulse of wanting to harm them. Reaction-formation can also be seen in abused children who run to the arms of the abuser, and in Stockholm Syndrome where the victims begin to empathize with their captors.

A barometer measures pressure. An *emotional barometer* measures the pressure of emotions on the being. Almost all pain and illness is barometric—indicating fluctuations in emotions. The body's health at any moment in time is the report card on the powerful unfelt emotions, and the sensation of isolation. Emotions are also the report card on the health of the relationships, especially the relationship with the *Self*—since there's no difference between others and the Self.

The physical body holds the states of relationships: the fear, anger, and rejection. However, due to ego and repression, the emotions attached to the states of the relationships, for the most part, remain unrecognized, until a symptom *suddenly appears*. The symptom tells us that something is bothering us because we can't, or won't, admit it to ourselves. The deeper Self is expressing itself through the body, as measured by the emotional pressure.

> In each of us there is another whom we do not know.
>
> Carl Jung

The complexity of the problem lies in accessing this unknown and unfelt side because the brain is sly when it comes to hiding shame. But we know that this side does exist from the vast successes over the past 100 years or so, of Josef Breuer, Franz Alexander, Sigmund Freud, Georg Groddeck, and the great Carl Jung, among others. Dr. Sarno will surely be placed in this same category because of how well he has blended body (medical science) and mind (psychology) together, much like Alexander and Groddeck. The great doctor was a keen observer of his patients, a rare trait among modern-day physicians. He was old-school medicine, a man who practiced what he preached, and put the patient first.

The division between the fields of mind and body is the paramount health problem today. Doctors treat bodies and psychologists treat minds. There are very few who will step into both arenas because neither feels comfortable crossing over into the other's territory. In addition, the specialized fields multiply the problems by dividing them into separate entities. But a person's mind and body are never separate. What happens in the mind is reflected in the body at all times; however, most modern health practitioners appear to only look at the body as the cause of the health problem.

The various fields have separated out the names of disorders like fibromyalgia, complex regional pain syndromes, reflex sympathetic dystrophies, repetitive stress disorders, pudendal neuralgias, plantar fasciitis, iliotibial band syndrome, piriformis syndrome, and chronic fatigue, in order to further study, and to further capitalize on them. Dr. Sarno brought these specialties back together into a more recognizable form by reintroducing the concept of psychosomatic disorders[9] to a world obsessed with treating symptoms. He did this by connecting emotions to physical symptoms. This, as he described it was, "rank heresy." Neither the health industry nor the sufferers wanted to hear it. The industry practitioners don't want to hear it because they feel they're doing more good than their predecessors had been doing for their clients, and they're also profiting. The sufferers don't want to hear that their physical symptoms are coming from their emotions for all the reasons laid out in this paean to Dr. Sarno.

Many of the symptoms we get, or have, result from an emotional process, as indicated by the emotional barometer. We are emotional beings, like it or not. Are there physical symptoms that are not from

---

[9] The older term "psychosomatic" is now referred to as mindbody.

a mindbody effect? Yes, of course. There are symptoms outside the mindbody realm, but most of the common health problems are from TMS; unfelt emotions. Sufferers aren't aware because they're being misled, and because many don't care to know. Most are content with the notion of a flawed body because it provides them cover from the very things their symptoms are hiding.

Due to a strong repressive tendency, many never realize they are holding such powerful emotions in the final form of tension. When pain strikes, many feel they've somehow hurt themselves from a certain movement, or as the result of a worn-out body part. But they've simply hit their personal repressive limit. The physical movement triggers the outpouring of energy and mental obsession, in the form of symptoms.

Almost all pain is initiated by a trigger, or triggers; the trigger more forcefully fortifies in the mind of the sufferer that he has indeed injured himself. Contrarily, TMS symptoms can also come from nowhere, in an acute attack, and they often do. The body will always be there when the mind needs help in hiding certain aspects of the Self. The body is the unconscious mind, as put forth by the late Candace Pert, PhD, in her work on the mindbody interaction. Candace Pert's pioneering work as a neuroscientist at the National Institutes of Mental Health proved the **mindbody connection** by demonstrating the connection between the brain and the body in what she called *molecules of emotion.*

'I've come to believe that virtually all illness, if not psychosomatic in foundation, has a definite psychosomatic component,' she wrote. The 'molecules of emotion,' she argued, 'run every system in our body,' creating a 'bodymind's intelligence' that is 'wise enough to seek wellness' without a great deal of high-tech medical intervention.

John Schwartz, New York Times,
Candace Pert, 67, Explorer of the Brain, Dies, 9/19/2013

Most people are unable to correlate the events in their lives with their newfound symptoms. However, if they look closer, many can trace the onset of their symptoms to a specific event in their life, or milestone plateau. If they're willing to accept TMS as the cause of their symptom, they will immediately think about what's going on in their life, and pay no heed to body.

The unpleasant symptoms are an emotional barometer, indicating hidden emotional pressure. But we have to know how to read the results. The barometer doesn't tell us where the pressure is coming from, only that it exists. It's up to the sufferer to piece the health puzzle together, and to find a solution to easing the pressure. That takes a great deal of reflective work, and courage to look beyond blaming the body. The body is the indicator of the problem, not the cause.

#4

Knowledge Therapy

> The most important factor in recovery is that the person must be made aware of what is going on; in other words, that the information provided is the 'penicillin' for this disorder ... I was mystified by the obvious importance of informing the patient what was going on. This was **knowledge therapy** ...
>
> John Sarno, MD, *Healing Back Pain*, p. 71

Dr. Sarno noticed—early on—that when he began explaining to his patients that their body was okay, and that their brain was fooling them with their pain to hide unconscious processes, some of them began to heal. A small fortunate few healed immediately, and the majority began the first steps on their personal healing journey. **The knowledge of TMS** began to transform their suffering into a much less dangerous prospect, and it began to set them free.

Much of the "knowledge healing mechanism" has to do with rendering the rage less threatening, behind the symptom. The unfelt rage behind pain is dangerous to the Self's desired image, so it's repressed at the behest of ego, and unrecognized within the individual's conscious self. The source of the rage may be eternally unknown; but somehow, the awareness of its existence through the emotional barometer—and in its purpose—renders it less dangerous to ego. *Reduced threat means reduced pain.*

The threat to ego comes from the fear of being and appearing out of control. As with phobias, confronting fear helps to dilute its authority. Deeper awareness brings a sense of order to the irrationality of the fear, similar to *exposure therapy* in phobias (reintegrating repressed emotions with current awareness), and anger is then tamed as a by-product. When we feel our body is broken, fear rises dramatically, and anger/rage is the social reaction to that fear.

Another reason that knowledge is therapeutic is that there's finally a reason for the amorphous suffering. After the person had spent years in doctors' offices, and perhaps tens of thousands of dollars with various health-practitioners, now finally—there's an answer that solves the mystery. The body is not broken! Whew—a great relief ... but with a new caveat! With this new knowledge, surrendering to truth suddenly means surrendering to yourself—to whom you are, and not to a broken body. This surrender is perceived by the deeper self to be even more painful.

It's also a pervasive reason that many people don't want to believe in TMS. It's much easier to surrender to a flawed body, than it is to see ourselves as we truly are, and to accept a life that has not gone as planned. To admit unhappiness is threatening to ego. It's less frightening (from ego's viewpoint) to believe that the body is broken, than to admit to a broken life—thus, *the great TMS controversy.*

Through repression, ego casts the unwanted into the body, to be stored. And so, this top-10 list of Dr. Sarno discoveries could easily be a top-11 list, if you consider that he identified a *repressive tension personality* (now called the Type-T). Many Type-Ts mistake their own personality for a Type-A, but the two are quite different.

Everyone has TMS. Everyone suffers from mindbody effects to varying degrees because we can never fully express ourselves at all times. The Type-T, however, appears to present with physical symptoms at a higher rate. The T is "Thee perfectionist," conscientious "goodist," gentle, kind, driven, detail-oriented worrier. These traits generate more powerful emotions, and therefore, more chronic symptoms.

This "awareness of personality" falls under *knowledge therapy* because most people aren't fully aware of how they're reacting to life. The "identifying of" this personality is part of the larger knowledge-healing package. Some sufferers are shocked to discover they're perfectionists. Some are incredulous to realize they're harboring powerful emotions. Others are astonished at the revelation that they're experiencing unconscious rage, while still others are disconcerted at being goodists. However, as knowledge is therapeutic, most of the sufferers begin to heal once they suddenly become aware of how they are **not reacting** to life.

It took a great observer to correlate these personality characteristics to the physical body symptoms, but an even greater observer to identify a narrower type of personality outside the commonly accepted personality types.

Beyond the reduction of the threat of rage, knowledge therapy also increases a *courage* factor. I've received several thousand emails from people who read *The Great Pain Deception*, and claimed it gave them courage to become more physical. The knowledge that movement will not further harm them is very empowering, and reduces fear. Hearing examples of others who have healed is also a powerful force, the proof of their success enables others to succeed.

Wherever there is fear, the counter response will be anger. And whenever fear and anger aren't as forcefully repressed, the mindbody's energy is freed for healing instead of repressing (hiding). The knowledge of what is occurring is the fundamental healing mechanism.

The knowledge that:

- The fear and rage are present
- The body is not broken, or failing
- The ego is controlling awareness
- The placebo fools, if the person is pleased

- The pain has a purpose
- There exists "another self" within
- TMS is harmless

This knowledge provokes a feeling of wellness, and renewed sense of control, which produces new neurotransmitters that transform the individual into a happier person—and energy skyrockets (if the brain doesn't use fatigue through the Symptom Imperative, discussed later: Spoiler Alert!).

There's also the knowledge healing mechanism, regarding "what not to do" in healing. Dr. Sarno wrote, "As long as he is preoccupied with what his body is doing, his symptoms will continue." Therefore, healing comes from never trying to heal—and in never obsessing on the body.

How can so-called "physical problems" be healed with the penicillin of knowledge? The shortest answer is that the physical body was never the cause of the physical symptoms. The symptoms and the body's defects had been spuriously correlated together in an *association error*.

Healing requires *two elements*. The first is to acquire the **knowledge** of how the anatomy, physiology, and psychology work together to form TMS. The second element is that the sufferer must *accept* that he has TMS. Without *acceptance*, all the knowledge in the universe won't help.

#3

Tension as the Cause of Pain

The key word in tension production is personality.

John Sarno, MD, *Mind Over Back Pain*, p. 50

One of the top three preeminent discoveries of the great doctor is that **tension is the cause** of most pain, and of countless other health problems. The multitude of various health problems that people experience every day are almost always caused by **tension**. Few health problems, except for injury, congenital defects, extreme dietary deficiencies, exposure to toxins, or pathological diseases, have anything to do with the body's structure. This is a revolutionary observation.

> **Revolutionary**: Latin, adjective; *radically new or innovative; outside or beyond established procedure and principles, a marked change.*

The healthcare industry has been heavily concentrating on fixing the body throughout the 19th and 20th centuries, instead of healing the person, and therefore, has rarely considered **tension** as the source of poor health. Many healthcare practitioners will say, "Of course tension can cause pain, and illness—we knew that!" But what they didn't know is that tension is causing **almost all** the pains, and a large majority of the illnesses. They also don't know that they—the practitioners themselves—are the primary cause of the epidemics because they aren't paying at-tension. And so, Dr. Sarno's tension observation wasn't just about unearthing the true cause and effects of ill-health—it was also a discovery of magnitude, blame, and faulty diagnoses.

We now know, from the great doctor's seminal work and astronomical success, that scientifically engineering the body into good health is causing, perpetuating, and exacerbating the problems. Under great stress, the brain desperately seeks diversion to the body, hoping that sufferers will look there; most sufferers fall into their brain's trap because they're told by their health practitioner that they have a body problem.

The "T" in TMS stands for tension. Nature has designed a body that knows how to repair itself; nature-ally. If the symptoms won't go away then they're likely driven by tension.

> Pain is, has been, and always will be a symptom. If it becomes severe and chronic, it is because that which is causing it is severe and has gone unrecognized. Chronicity, in the case of these pain syndromes, is a function of faulty diagnosis.

John Sarno, MD, *Healing Back Pain*, p. 130

Generally speaking, there's nothing wrong with the hands and feet, shoulders and knees, hips, neck, and back. The body's core does not need to be strengthened or aligned properly. Spinal discs cannot slip in and out of place. One leg longer than the other, or one hip higher than another, does not cause pain (beyond the belief that it does). The body doesn't need to be stretched, aligned, strengthened, cut, injected, or fixed in any way—when stress-induced tension is the culprit. The very acts of poking, prodding, stretching, stabbing, cutting, realigning, and talking about body must be stopped.

Sources of Tension

When it comes to mindbody health issues, people often use the words stress and tension interchangeably because they're closely related—coexisting.

Stress occurs psychologically when we don't get what we want. Stress is the difference between "what we wanted" versus "what we just got."

Stress is a "short on" problem: short on time, short on patience, short on money, short on brains, short on pleasure. Therefore, psychological stress occurs from a *negative perception* of events. When we think we want some specific thing—but in our judgment—we got something else, or nothing at all, we become stressed.

Tension is the body's physical response to that stress. Stress is *perceived* within the *mind*, and tension is *real* within the *body*. TMS is a real physical mindbody effect that begins as a perception within, and permeates the corporeal body as crippling pain, illness, and fatigue.

Confusion in the understanding of TMS is a result of the interactions of *ego, placebo*, and the *Symptom Imperative*.[10] Sadly, one of the leading reasons people refuse to accept that they themselves are experiencing a mindbody effect is that it insults them. I hear it virtually every day, "You are insulting my intelligence with this nonsense." They then go on to live lives of suffering because they can't get beyond their *ego's perception*—and because they've experienced prior temporary placebo results in healing. The placebo and the Symptom Imperative shifting make them believe that they once had a physical structural problem, when they didn't. A placebo **forces the symptom to shift forms** if the reasons for the tension still remain, resulting from the perception of events—as seen by the personality.

Consequently, there begins a string of unfortunate events that all begin with a perception. When adding to this the element that it all occurs outside of awareness, the end result is confusion, denial,

---

[10] The Symptom Imperative: the brain causes the symptoms to shift around in the body.

and an even greater controversy. Although TMS is not imagined, the process begins in the mind, and the body reacts accordingly, altering immunity, and autonomic functions. The presence of symptoms reveals a state of dis-ease: *an unnatural state of ease and mind.*

Ease: Old French, noun; *freedom from pain or trouble, comfort of body or mind.*

Dr. Sarno contended that you don't always have to eliminate the tension to heal, but it certainly helps if you can. The idea in tension reduction is to change the perception of the need to fight or flee to one of **surrendering**, and the body will not react as strongly. It's imperative to also change the perception of the pain itself from believing it's doing damage to the body, to understanding that it's only diverting awareness to the body, as well as sending a deeper message of dis-ease.

Stress isn't always from a false perception because there may indeed be imminent danger. We can't entirely rid ourselves of fear or we would walk into oncoming traffic, jump off buildings, pet poisonous animals, or get married without prenuptial agreements.

In modern-day life we abuse and misuse the stress function within the fight/flight survival mechanism, from false perceptions of danger. We no longer need to run from tigers, or hunt for food. Today's tigers are the bosses, competitors, Smiths and Joneses, and crosses of *self-imposed demands.* The tension primarily emanates from the demands we place on ourselves to not only be good, and then to be better … but to be perfect!

The Out-of-Control Train of Events

The conflicted mind leading to health disorders begins with a perception that we didn't get what we thought we wanted, or weren't as good as we thought we should have been. Stress from that perception is then transduced into tension in the body. The tension then disrupts the harmonious state of ease and balance within the mindbody, manifesting as pain and disease. These states are normal in acute phases, as danger comes and goes throughout the act of surviving. However, perfection, and never ending self-demands, fueled by guilt and shame, won't allow the state of fight/flight to disengage. The mindbody never has a chance to fall back into ease, and poor health permeates the body. As tension becomes chronic, and if not countered with some sort of soothing, its effects can range from unpleasant, to crippling, to death. And it all begins with "want."

Want: Old Norse, verb; *to wish, need, crave, demand, or desire.*

Tension follows wanting. Sufferers are unknowingly doing it to themselves, beyond their awareness—wishing to be good people, desiring to get along, needing to be better, craving for pleasure, and wanting to do what is right. Personality heavily influences stress levels that generate tension, that cause the physical problems identified by Dr. Sarno.

Personality is the major factor in tension production, and in its chronicity. Of course, tension can come from any number of life-threatening scenarios, and traumas, that have little to do with personality. But if you add trauma and perceived emotional abandonment to a conscientious/driven personality, the end result is a very unhealthy person with dangerous tension levels.

Personality contains the patterns of behavioral characteristics, corrupted memory, and the summation of traits of the individual that help determine whether an event is perceived as bad, or stressful. It also determines how much a person will fight to survive, and which survival method will be used. The Type-T uses **thinking** as a primary survival tool. They often live their lives in their heads as stress-thinkers, ruminators, dreamers, what-iffers, and procrastinators.

Thinking (mental calculating) drives brainwave activity into a heightened Beta-state of awareness. The more mental scenarios the sufferer runs through, the more Beta is intensified. Beta brainwave activity is associated with the highest number of hospital visits. Tension comes from stress, and stress comes not only from real danger (wanting to survive), but also from perceived danger, wanting, and **thinking**. Clearing the mind of danger, desires, wanting, and mental chatter eases tension, and has been referred to as **meditation**. Meditation does not necessarily heal pain, but it can be a great tool in reversing the cacophonous mental state that gives rise to tension, especially if the meditation takes the sufferer into the pain, and not away from it.

Thinking is the opposite of doing. French philosopher Émile Chartier wrote, "To think is to say no." Doing means action and involvement, and with repetitive action often comes reduced tension. Thinking can lead to hesitation, frustration, anticipation, and worry—leading to tension, and TMS.

 While Beta brain waves are important for effective functioning throughout the day, they also can translate into stress, anxiety, and restlessness. The voice of Beta can be described as being that nagging little inner critic that gets louder the higher you go into range. Therefore, with a majority of adults operating in Beta, it's little surprise that stress is today's most common health problem.

FinerMinds.com

Dr. Sarno proved that tension wreaks mindbody havoc. It causes back pain, foot and hand pain, leg and knee pain, shoulder and arm pain. It ignites ulcers and migraines, activates face, tooth, and jaw pain. It blurs vision and distorts hearing, and irritates the skin. It disrupts autonomic activity, causing disharmony in the functions of breathing, bloodflow, sleep, and digestion. Tension affects the immune system and how the body heals from infections, and repairs itself after surgery, and injury.

But there's more. Tension creates odd body sensations, electrical snapping, cold waves, pins and needles, thumping, burning, dizziness, pressure, numbness, stiffness, buzzing, and stabbing. If tension remains chronic, it leads to adrenal exhaustion, fatigue, and immune suppression. It can cause the body to attack itself, inducing autoimmune reactions, and heart attacks. The list of physical problems that tension can create is too large to list because it's infinite. And yet, few professionals are taking this into account when diagnosing patients. Instead, they are focusing on fixing the body.

Health practitioners are now warning people to limit smartphones, and electronic devices to prevent text-necks, and to be careful of slim line jeans, lifting wrong, wearing the wrong shoes, sitting in comfy chairs, and of sleeping on soft mattresses. They warn of crooked spines, weak bodies, and poor work habits. They hand out bad advice every day—and that advice creates more tension because stress rises higher when anxious people are constantly worrying about "doing things in the correct manner."

Tension soars dramatically when the sufferer is told that something is physically wrong. Dr. Sarno turned the tables on such insidious notions with his work in understanding the role of tension in pain, and illness.

The various health disciplines interested in the back have succeeded in creating an army of the partially disabled in this country with their medieval concepts of structural damage and injury as the basis of back pain.

John Sarno, MD, *Healing Back Pain*, p. 79

Stress resulting from perceptions, mental calculating, misguided beliefs, and bad advice leads to tension-induced health problems. The body always seems to get blamed, but humans simply aren't that weak. However, as society is currently wired, it appears content on treating the body instead of healing the individual. Watch a half hour of TV health commercials and see where the priorities lie. If we would only focus our energy and efforts on how to live, instead of trying to figure out how to not die, we would be dramatically healthier, and happier.

In his prolific career, the great doctor proved the effects that tension has on health. As a medical doctor, he diagnosed sufferers, but as a teacher, he helped them heal. He stated that he didn't "heal" anyone, that they healed themselves with knowledge, and belief. A large part of that knowledge was the awareness of the existence of unconscious tension, and in accepting it as the cause of their pain.

#2

A Favor by the Brain: Protective Mechanism

 It was a psychoanalyst colleague, Dr. Stanley Coen, who suggested in the course of our working on a medical paper together that the role of the pain syndrome was not to express the hidden emotions but to prevent them from becoming conscious ... it is intended to focus one's attention on the body instead of the mind ... the mark of a good camouflage is that it will not be recognized for what it is, that no one will know that something is being hidden.

John Sarno, MD, *Healing Back Pain*, p. 48

Dr. Sarno wrote of the now internationally famous Helen, who was bedridden and "paralyzed with pain." At 47, she had remembered being molested by her father when she was a little girl, and had joined an incest support group to try to heal her emotional wounds. As she entered the support group, her symptoms began to worsen. She couldn't understand why she was getting worse but her husband insightfully pointed out, "You're talking about forty years of repressed anger." His words suddenly triggered an emotional catharsis as she cried harder than she had ever cried in her life: as she described, "out-of-control tears." She began blurting out words such as "let me die," "I feel sick," "I'm so afraid," "please take care of me." From that point, Helen described her pain leaving her like a pipeline from her lower back through her eyes, pouring out of her—and her pain ended. Her pain initially began to increase—as it often does—to prevent certain emotions from entering consciousness. In the end, her surrendering to the truth set her free, as her pain had no more purpose—having only existed to suppress her unconscious rage.

> Most pain and illness exist to protect the sufferer, which is why they often don't want to believe in TMS. They reject it outright because it's protecting them from what's painful beneath their awareness.

TMS physical pain is an emotional memory that can't be let go, the sting of which is too threatening for ego to admit to. It would be nice if we could throw those memories away as fast as the first AARP card we get in the mail. But it doesn't work that way. We hold fear, anger, sorrow, and resentment in our bodies, to protect us from experiencing (feeling) the full brunt of the pain of those emotions, and to reduce their threat to ego. They're held in the body as unpleasant physical sensations in order to help maintain the *persona*—to outwardly appear as if all is going well. Ego is central to the problem of ongoing suffering, as the body takes the heat for trying to appear cool.

This is the *second best observation* of the great doctor, yet another centerpiece of his life's work. Most pains and illnesses are psychological defense mechanisms—created by the brain, at the direction of ego—in order to divert the sufferer's attention to the body, and away from ego-threatening thoughts and emotions. But note that he gave credit to his colleague Dr. Coen for the primary insight. This is also part of Dr. Sarno's success, and mystique. He was a consummate professional; labeled by Forbes Magazine in 2012 as "America's Best Doctor."

Dr. Sarno has no idea he's a rock star. That's why he's cool—he doesn't know it. From East to West, and North to South, people around the world admire him and love him because they healed from his insight, and his courage. But they also **admire how he did it**. The way in which a message is delivered is often as important as the message itself, especially regarding something as sensitive to ego as TMS. He simply stated what he was seeing. He wasn't dogmatic or arrogant, and never wanted to play a blame game. His goal was to educate, to help.

A huge part of his success results from *his own personality.* Countless people, from professionals to laymen, were healed with his work. Many of them get very emotional when they talk about what he did for them. Some met him, while others followed and watched, and learned from him. He had the "It" factor that can't be defined. And whatever It was—It worked! He was sincere, humble, professional, courageous, and correct. People long for direction, especially when they're suffering, and they will follow confidence to the gates of heaven. His *confidence* in what he was observing, as a scientist, helped sufferers to heal.

When you look at the many surveys throughout history, regarding "the most attractive traits," whether it's in males or females, the most attractive personality trait reported by those surveyed is almost always **confidence**. People are drawn toward people who walk straight and narrow paths, probably because they themselves are confused and lacking direction. Then, when a person comes along with proof of truth, who is confident in his or her own path, people will follow that light.

In the end, it is **belief** and **acceptance** that heal people from TMS: not science or medicine. If people believe their body is broken, they suffer. If they accept that their body is okay, they tend to heal. The great doctor's confidence allowed people to see that their bodies were okay, and if they accepted that notion, they healed.

Frustrated with his prior results, he wanted to help somehow. His courage was instrumental to his successes. Dr. Coen suggested that most pains were diversions, but Dr. Sarno went out and proved it. Dr. Coen wasn't the one riding the edge, being mocked, pushing the message. Dr. Sarno wrote the books, conveyed the points, and weathered the heat. Just as Freud didn't create psychoanalysis—but mainstreamed it—Dr. Sarno may not have originated the idea of "symptom as distraction," but he observed it, pulled it into a concept, and passed it to the people. He ran with this hypothesis for the rest of his career and it proved to be correct.

Pain is a defense against Truth. The "protective favors" of pain and dis-ease, by the brain, help the sufferer avoid painful thoughts and emotions, but it also has a downside to it. As anyone who has ever healed knows, the worst thing you can do is to try to help someone else recover from their own suffering. Most people see TMS as a weakness, but it isn't. So on one hand, the brain's favor helps the sufferer avoid dangerous thoughts and emotions by diverting awareness to the body—but simultaneously, the brain's scheme won't allow the person to ever heal.

You can't heal until you recognize that you indeed possess strong emotions—and accept that they are causing your symptoms. The TMS protective mechanism by the brain can be seen as a crutch that keeps the person walking, but crippled. The very reason she refuses to believe in TMS is also the reason she has her pain: *refusing to see herself as she truly is.* This is a top-two observation.

#1

The Symptom Imperative

> Well, Jayne, it just goes to show ya, it's always somethen. If it's not one thing … it's another.
>
> Roseanne Roseannadanna, "Saturday Night Live"

I told the great doctor on the phone in April of 2012, that I believed this was his greatest discovery. His observation of what he called **The Symptom Imperative** answered so many of our health problems. Until that point, people were simply labeled as "unlucky in health." A sufferer may have had neck surgery, then shoulder surgery, followed by back, foot, knee, or hand surgery—and then may have subsequently experienced ulcers, sleeplessness, anxiety, or (m)any other types of health issues. **The Symptom Imperative is about need.**

Where once their family and friends, or society, would have considered them to be physically unlucky—drowning in their own genetic cesspool—we now know from the good doctor's Symptom Imperative observation, that this person only had **one problem: TMS.** That "one problem" was bounding around in them taking on alternating forms, appearing as a variety of health issues, giving medical chase—eluding proper diagnoses—**demanding attention.** In this case, the wrong attention is administered to the patient, which is attention to the body symptoms, and no attention is given to the cause, which is the emotions.

All the unlucky ones need to do is become aware of the unfelt emotional process, and accept it, and most of their health problems will fade. Once they discover how they're reacting to life, or more precisely, how they are NOT reacting to life, they've begun their healing expedition. How far they travel on their new journey depends on many interrelated factors, such as full belief, ego control, depth of fear, heat of anger, coolness of confidence, capacity for courage, degree of desire, and need for the symptoms.

The TMS message is not anti-doctor, nor anti-medicine. We need good healers, we need more great doctors; but it needs to be re-emphasized that it is the physicians who are unwittingly adding to many of the health problems by telling sufferers that they have physical body problems, when they don't. Few were paying attention until the great doctor published his findings.

Symptoms are: *Changes, such as, swelling, redness, itching, pins and needles, hot, cold, numbness, electrical snapping, weakness, anxiety, and pain.*

Imperative: *Something that demands attention.*

The Symptom Imperative means: *A change in the physical body that demands attention. However, "the thing" demanding the attention is not the body, it's the unmet needs.*

No matter how many surgeries, healing techniques, physical therapies, medications, or therapeutic modalities of any kind that a person receives—if the **need** for the physical symptom still exists, a symptom will keep popping up; this is necessary to maintain the individual's belief that something is wrong with his body. This is the essence of The Symptom Imperative phenomenon.

The Symptom Imperative, SI, encapsulates all the great doctor's nine best discoveries above into a single health dénouement. It epitomizes the concept of TMS. I believe this is Dr. Sarno's greatest contribution to the understanding of health, and deserving of a Nobel Prize in Medicine. I believe it because I lived it, and have seen thousands of people jumping through the same painful hoops: unsuccessfully trying to solve their many agonizing health issues, futilely trying to scientifically treat their body into good health. I've also seen thousands heal upon recognition of the SI.

Example 1: She has back surgery—she soon develops sleeplessness.

Because of the placebo effect, she believed her back was healed; but it wasn't, because there was nothing that needed healing. Her back pain was an effect of her unconscious tension, from her unknown psychological conflict. Since her conflict still exists, it must necessarily shift somewhere else in order to continue to hold her attention. With her newfound sleeplessness, she now feels that she has developed a new health problem, but it's only her old problem in a new form, demanding old attention. Her back pain was never coming from her spinal structure; but having been deeply pleased by her surgery, and by her surgeon's confidence in the procedure, her back feels "somewhat" better. Her deeper-self believed surgery worked, and so her symptom shifts somewhere else as her brain creates a new distraction; a new obsession for her to worry about. **Her emotions hide behind her worry, not the symptom itself.**

Her brain creates sleeplessness so that she can worry about something new, now that her brain is no longer worrying about her back pain. If she doesn't buy into the worry or concern over her new sleep problem, it won't stick around. Her obsession is the force that keeps her new symptom alive. If she had no doubts about her new problem being serious, or if she wasn't concerned that it was even a problem, her brain would not keep generating the sleeplessness. It would eventually give up its strategy and shift once again until it could find something else that concerned her. Once it finds something that she **fears**—there it stays, as her new TMS, her brain's new gift to her.

Her muted rage over self-imposed demands to be good, and to always do what is right, generates the need for her ego to divert her awareness to her body—to prevent her from emitting, and seeing, a side of herself that she has no wish to be. Her worry is the mechanism that determines which symptoms will be utilized by her brain. If she doesn't fear her new symptom as being real (a health problem), her brain will continue to "shift symptoms" until it finds a place (symptom) that causes her to fear a serious problem. At that point, her brain has found a new fear where she can hide her emotions. It isn't the symptom her brain hides her anger behind, it's the worry of the symptom—the obsession.

Example 2: He has knee surgery—soon his other knee begins to hurt.

He feels he has placed too much pressure on his knee while the surgery-knee was recovering. But that's not what happened. His shrewd brain simply shifted the diversion to his second knee in its fervent need to sustain some form of distraction. Any pressure he may have been placing on it during convalescence was a **trigger**. When his doctor tells him that he should indeed be worried about his second knee because it, too, has "meniscus tearing and arthritis," he then begins to experience a new round of The Symptom Imperative. As long as he is unaware of what is occurring, he will spend his time, energy, and focus trying to heal what he feels is a body problem. But his health issues are only one problem; the other problem is that his brain is incessantly demanding a diversion.

At this point he may have discovered TMS, and may now understand that his first knee never required surgery to heal. However, this other knee pain feels "different" than his surgery-knee. This time he knows the pain is real! Ahhh ... but the brain is sly when utilizing The Symptom Imperative. It not only changes the form of the symptom, it also **alters the sensation** to keep the fear of the body symptom strong. The more structural the brain can make the symptom feel, the better it serves as a force of distraction. The brain learned from the first time around that the sensation it had presented in the first knee "wasn't good enough" to maintain fear because he believed the surgery actually worked: a new Symptom Imperative begins.

The more threatening the thoughts and emotions driving the symptoms, the more frantically the brain will work to maintain fear. The brain's intent is always to create worry. The more worry given to the body, the less attention will be paid to the unwanted thoughts and emotions.

Example 3: She has rotator cuff surgery—she falls into deep depression.

Because her belief is powerful, her shoulder feels better after surgery. However, this time, instead of her brain shifting diversion back to her body, it acquiesces and caves in to the emotion that was generating the shoulder pain. It shifted from symptom as a diversion to the psychological need for the diversion. It steps directly to the edge of the event horizon, the depression.

Depression is often the cause of the need for body symptoms. It is the most frightening of sensations; so much so, that whenever it looms the brain will desperately seek ways to create physical manifestations to divert the mind's eye from the darkness. However, the depression itself can be seen as a breakthrough (a matter of perception). The brain has finally abandoned its strategy of fooling the individual into thinking there are health problems. Its new emotional diversion can be viewed as a "changing strategy," or it can be seen as an emotional decline, as though the brain is giving up. Life is a matter of perception, just as happiness is a choice. From my experience, the last stage before healing is the emergence of the emotions behind the symptoms, which is a positive step, not a decline.

Accurate perception is essential to healing. Commonly, after learning about TMS, a sufferer's pain begins to spread. They then become frantic, thinking they're getting worse. They need to understand that they're winning! Their brain doesn't like that they're becoming aware, and so it panics by spreading the symptoms in order to maintain fear. The proper perception of events is at the Rubicon of determining stress levels, and eventual outcomes of good or bad.

The Symptom Imperative employs **conscious awareness**—the struggle for conscious thought within a conflicted mind, driven by the fervent desire to hide fear and shame. The SI can take an infinite variety of forms, including back pain, migraines, vision problems, anxiety, skin disorders, numbness, tingling, frequent urination, weakness, fatigue, pressure, electrical snapping, coldness, irritable bowel, painful bladder, swelling, stiffness, and odd sensations like a burning mouth. And it can also shift back to the psychological realm: to anxiety, rage, sadness, and depression. The list is infinite because the brain has carte blanche to create whatever it has authority over to help the person cope with life—to avoid the unwanted, with the sole purpose of shunning rejection.

The power that the mind wields is over the body itself—the two being one—and its **mechanisms for creating diversions** are often memories (remembering old wounds), awareness (of body malformations), and observation (memes—catching others' problems). However, a symptom can often appear as spontaneous.

The above examples aren't merely examples; they actually happened. These people healed once they recognized they had been fooled by their brain into thinking they had a physical problem.

Beyond the Symptom Imperative

Now if a pain sufferer eventually gets to that deeper point of awareness, where he understands that his body is okay—and from this new knowledge frees himself of pain and illness, but **still has fear**—his focus and obsessive worry **will still need** an outlet. He may have deeply integrated the concept of TMS, and no longer obsesses on his body, and has dealt with the anxiety and depression. However, if fear has a dominating presence, the brain will demand continued diversion away from darkness.

At this point, awareness will shift into **The Shadow Imperative**.

- The former neck-pain sufferer **now** develops food **paranoia**
- The former shoulder-pain sufferer **now** becomes **agoraphobic**
- The former smoker **now** shifts to projection: **judging** others
- The former alcoholic **now** shifts to sugars and caffeine, for **stimulation**
- The former knee-pain sufferer is now obsessed with exercise and training

If there's no life purpose, or deeper passion, the need for a diversion doesn't end when the Symptom Imperative no longer serves to divert worry. Obsessions continue as long as fear is a driving force. The ouroboros cycle continues as long as there is a deep **spiritual yearning**—the need for a purpose more important than life, beyond the mind's governance of the physical senses.

Fear is the great motivator. Running from it feeds it, keeping it alive, allowing it to morph into various physical and psychological forms. The only thing that satisfies the hunger of fear is **surrender**—to who you are, to what already is, to Truth.

Jung's definition of the shadow: "The thing a person has no wish to be."

Carl Jung, *Collective Works*, vol. 16[11]

Imperative: *Still demands attention.*

Everyone possesses a shadow. The shadow contains all our fears and perceived weaknesses. It comprises all our emotions and impulses of power-desire, sexual-cravings, greed-temptations, envy-wants—and threatening-rage. The shadow elements within the psyche run contrary to what we deem to be socially acceptable, and so they're denied expression by the Self. We simply don't want to believe that we have certain unsavory aspects, and that we could ever possess certain thoughts and desires. And we certainly don't want others to see these traits in us, so we deny their existence altogether. From this denial, the Self becomes conflicted. What we think we are, and what we really are, is constantly vying for expression. The goal is to integrate these traits—into wholeness—and for the mind divided to become one with it-Self, through **individuation**.

Individuation: *Coming to terms with the opposites within your Self. Uniting the unconscious with the conscious, becoming your potential, what you always were.*

The urge to individuation gathers together what is scattered ... in this way our existence as separate beings, our former ego-nature, is abolished, the circle of consciousness is widened, and because the paradoxes have been made conscious, the sources of conflict are dried up.

Carl Jung, *Collective Works*, vol. 11

---

[11] Collected Works of C. G. Jung, Volume 16 paragraph 470, Princeton University Press.

The individuation into wholeness comes through surrendering to perceived imperfections. The imbalances in mindbody labeled "pain and illness" are most often effects of denying unwanted thoughts and emotions that are considered as being too threatening. The conflict within Self creates the vast majority of health problems, as Dr. Sarno proved beyond any "shadow" of doubt.

Seeing ourselves as perfect and flawless greatly affects psychic-balance because the total-Self knows it isn't true. The deeper-self understands that these darker forces exist, and not only wants to admit their existence, but even more dangerous, to act on them. The shame of admitting to fear, rage, want, and desire is the reason for the mind's conflict because the mind is divided between what it wants—*and*—what it has deemed to be unacceptable to others. The ego is the referee in this battle of repression versus expression.

Dr. Sarno asserted at the end of his 50-year career that, "These people are suffering because they want to be good people." They want to do what is right. They want to take care of those around them. They want to keep everyone happy because they feel they should—*yet simultaneously*—they don't care about those things. He stated that this type of goodist behavior is great for society, but unfortunately, the shadow-self wants nothing to do with goodist behavior. It is angered by ego's notion of pretending.

Pretending: Latin, *prae "before" tendere "to stretch;"* to *deceive, to feign, to make falsely believe.*

Common Threads of Deception

One of the revered gurus of Nondualism, Nisargadatta Maharaj, had his life transformed when his guru taught him, "You are not what you take yourself to be." And Lesson 166, in *A Course In Miracles*, similarly implies: *we are not who we are pretending to be.*

 This is your chosen self, the one you made as a replacement for reality. This is the self you savagely defend against all reason, every evidence, and all the witnesses with proof to show this is not you. You heed them not. You go on your appointed way, with eyes cast down lest you might catch a glimpse of truth, and be released from self-deception, and set free.

"A Course in Miracles," Lesson: 166

One of the most basic tenets of the ancient art of Ayurvedic healing is that people become sick and pained because "they can't show their true faces." When we separate from Truth we suffer.

This all fits perfectly with Freud's concept of *superego*; the aspect of the psyche that holds all the **moral standards** and **ideals** of "how we feel we should act," in accordance with society's wishes. The main action of the superego is to suppress any desires of the true Self that are deemed socially unacceptable. Superego strives for perfection; it doesn't care what the person wants, or about the current realities. It is a false-Self—built to suppress, and deny.

The philosophy of a false-Self also exists within Carl Jung's work on the **persona**. The word *personality* derives from the Latin word, *persona*, which means "mask." Masks are worn for both deception and protection:

- To protect self-image by preventing others from seeing true aspects of our-Self

- To deceive others into thinking that we are who we are pretending to be

Within the processes of deception and protection, the Self becomes even more conflicted **when it begins to believe** that it is what it is pretending to be. At this point, ego has sold out to superego. In the pretending, the sufferer loses the notion of Self: its full potential, good health, and real happiness.

I've had thousands of people email me after reading *The Great Pain Deception,* to tell me they began seeing deeper into themselves. For the first time in their lives, they became aware of aspects of themselves they had been denying, and they began to heal. But it takes great courage to look into the darkness. We don't find what we don't look for, and we don't look for what we don't want to see. We don't even know to look if we don't know something is missing. In this sense the physical suffering is a blessing. All those who healed were ready to see themselves, to become whole.

The butterfly sheds its restraints once it's ready to reveal its beauty. Those who aren't ready to shine, continue to defend physical problems as the basis for their suffering. But that's okay. Everyone comes to truth in their own time. Healing is metaphoric for "readiness," and for acceptance. In the denial of truth, the shadow becomes a destructive force through its habitual need to be heard. What is truth? It's who we already are—it's repeatable, like love.

> A man who is possessed by his Shadow is always standing in his own light and falling into his own traps … living below his own level.

Carl Jung, *Archetypes*, pg. 23

As long as denial is used as a shield, the sufferer will run through the gauntlet of health problems, year by year, perhaps for life—until she finally accepts that her body is okay, and that she has been fooled by her brain into believing her body is defective. The medical techniques employed will only chase her problems around, never solving anything. The proof is that despite possessing the most advanced medical techniques in the history of humankind, the pain epidemics are worsening: they're not getting better. The human body is very strong. It isn't failing and in need of constant repair. It knows how to heal, if ego allows for it.

Negotiating with the shadow is painful because people are shocked to discover who they are, with weaknesses, frailties, shortcomings, peculiarities, defects, and with what Jung called "demonic dynamism." We are capable of great bad ... or great good if light is chosen over dark.

The rage and fear driving the physical symptoms come from two major sources:

1) **The shadow**: All emotional pain is cast into the shadow. The shadow also contains all the answers to the problems but is reluctant to give them up because of shame. The unconscious will influence the conscious, but it needs to be enticed out, and recognized.

2) **The daily stressors**: These sources of stress over-stimulate the sympathetic nervous system. The daily-life stressors are blamed for poor health, but as the cause of most pains and illnesses, their role is actually far less. Almost all TMS pain flows from enduring childhood anger—as daily life gets screened through the prism of the hurt child. As children, they either never learned how to express fear and anger, or were never allowed to express it. Now as adults, they push through their responsibilities with ego screening events through corrupted memories of fear of abandonment and low self-esteem, driven by the "need to be perfect" in order to overcome perceived weaknesses. This occurs to avoid **rejection**, since our deepest need is to **feel connected**.

Our greatest strengths we have today were once weaknesses that we fought to overcome. Hence, the shadow is an integral part of growth. If we don't want to be something, i.e., shadow, we grow away from it, in any way we can. The shadow then is our **inner gold** that helps us to become more peaceful, happier. We can't become whole until we first see that we're imperfect. There's no recognition of light without darkness.

> The shadow is a tight passage, a narrow door, whose painful constriction no one is spared who goes down to the deep well.
>
> Carl Jung

Ask any scientist what truth is and their answer will most likely be that truth is "repeatable through measurement." By that definition, TMS is immensely repeatable, and so true. However, it's not measurable, only observable. Dr. Sarno's The Mindbody Syndrome is one of the greatest observations in medical history. And his Symptom Imperative paints the overall picture by revealing how all the medical techniques for pain, including the new medications, are only serving the brain in its great deception.

As long as sufferers seek physical solutions for emotional expressions, the *Symptom Imperative* will be available, in every form. Beyond that, if the individual integrates the concept of TMS, and no longer fears the body symptoms—but still has psychic conflict—the *Shadow Imperative* will be present to continue to divert awareness from fear, and to help with personal growth, in the expansion of spirit.

When the sufferer is not who he or she is pretending to be, the mind will be divided in conflict between what it wants and what it can't have—*and*—in what it knows to be true versus how it's currently acting (cognitive dissonance).

The great doctor changed the world with these observations, but the world hasn't become aware of it ... yet. I believe these 10 discoveries to be his most wonderful gifts to humanity. The merit of each will be debated for decades to come. But to anyone who has benefited from his work, the importance of these findings can never be overstated.

The distinguished Spanish painter, sculptor, and poet, Pablo Picasso, said, "The meaning of life is to find your gift. The purpose of life is to give it away." And so, Dr. Sarno, the TMS physicians, TMS therapists and counselors, TMS consultants and coaches, TMS authors, and former TMS sufferers continue to try to help as many as are willing to listen, to give the gift away. The resistance is strong, but like a slow-burning fire, the light expands across the darkness revealing truth along the way. The only thing standing in the way is ignorance: *a lack of awareness.* There's only so much people can do in one lifetime. Dr. Sarno did what he could, and more.

I've tried on several occasions to encapsulate what the great doctor did in his career, in order to explain it to people who are curious, or who are short on patience. The answer that I come up with keeps changing. But I've currently reached the conclusion that **he empowered people**. We are not helpless/hapless victims of our bodies. We control our health far more than we realize. We don't have to suffer, we can heal; but it takes courage, and desire.

Dr. John Sarno changed current thinking by uprooting a false paradigm in medicine with his **observations** and **courage**, against a backlash of criticism and cynicism. Some scorned him, while others mocked the joy of those who benefited from his gifts. But no matter how much the Grinch-like TMS naysayers try to steal the presence of peace and happiness, they can't. Those who healed are forever changed for the better by a man who was the essence of a true healer. Dr. Sarno had the career of ten doctors—plus two!

Also by Steve Ozanich

The Great Pain Deception:
Faulty Medical Advice Is Making Us Worse

Back Pain
Permanent Healing:
Understanding the
Myths, Lies, and Confusion

on YouTube at
TMS Healing Wall of Victory - The Great Pain Deception

SteveOzanich.com

Steve Ozanich, a mindbody health consultant, penned *The Great Pain Deception* based on his own experience, the work of John Sarno, MD, and ten years of intensive research. Its success in educating the public led him to pen a follow up book in 2016, entitled, *Back Pain: Myths, Lies, and Confusion.*

Over the past 16 years, Ozanich has literally taught thousands of people how to heal themselves. He earned three degrees from Youngstown State University: AAS, BSAS, and MBA, with four consecutive Distinguished Student Awards from the Dean of The Williamson School of Business.

In addition to being a mindbody health consultant, the Ohio-based Ozanich is a health blogger with JenningsWire, a health lecturer, personal fitness trainer, acoustic guitar player, and golf-swing coach.

Made in the USA
Middletown, DE
15 January 2017